PILATES FOR SENIORS

Step by step guide to safe and effective exercise

Dr. Bryant D Baldwin

The trademarks that are used are without any consent, and the publication of the trademark is without permission or backing by the trademark owner. All trademarks and brands within this book are for clarifying purposes only and are owned by the owners themselves, not affiliated with this document.

Table Of Content

Scan this Area to access bonus

INTRODUCTION

A Pilates Overview

Pilates is a type of exercise that emphasizes core stability while also enhancing flexibility and balance. A popular kind of exercise for people of all ages and fitness levels, it was created in the early 20th century by German physical trainer Joseph Pilates.

Seniors are one demographic that Pilates can be particularly beneficial to. Our bodies experience changes as we get older, which can make it harder to be physically active and maintain excellent health. Falls and other accidents are more likely when muscles and joints are weak and inflexible.

Pilates is a low-impact exercise that is both safe and efficient for senior citizens. The slow, deliberate movements emphasize using the body's natural resistance to increase strength and flexibility. Seniors benefit from this since it lowers their risk of injury and makes daily activities more comfortable and easy for them.

Benefits of Pilates for older adults

1. Pilates aims to balance the body by improving posture, bolstering the core muscles, and improving flexibility and motor control. Instead of focusing on quantity, the goal is to improve movement quality and build a solid mental-physical connection.

2. Pilates emphasizes breathing, proper alignment, and controlled movements in

addition to preventing injuries and enhancing overall health and well-being.

3. Seniors who practice Pilates can benefit from increased strength, flexibility, and balance as well as better coordination and balance.

4. The emphasis on deliberate, precise movement enhances the body's ability to communicate with the brain, which can help lower the chance of falling.

5. Seniors who practice Pilates can also benefit from better alignment and posture. The core muscles, which are in charge of supporting the spine and upholding proper posture, are the emphasis of the exercises. Seniors can improve their posture and lower their risk of back pain and other related problems by exercising these muscles.

Additionally, seniors' mental health may benefit from Pilates. It is a type of mind-body workout that can lessen stress and enhance general well-being. The contemplative and calming nature of the slow, regulated motions can boost mood and lessen anxiety.

In conclusion, seniors can exercise safely and effectively with Pilates. It is low-impact and can enhance balance, flexibility, coordination, posture, and alignment, as well as general health.

The value of continuing to be active as we age

As we get older, being active is crucial to maintaining our general health and well-being. Regular exercise can lengthen life, enhance mental health, and help prevent chronic diseases.

Age-related physical changes in our bodies can increase our risk of developing chronic conditions including osteoporosis, diabetes, and heart disease. By strengthening bones, regulating weight, and enhancing cardiovascular health, regular exercise can lower the risk of developing these diseases. Regular physical activity can further improve cholesterol and blood pressure levels, which lowers the risk of heart disease.

Physical exercise can help lessen the signs of depression and anxiety, which is good for mental health. Endorphins are brain chemicals that are released during exercise and which can elevate mood and lessen stress. Additionally, physical activity helps enhance the quality of sleep, which is frequently disturbed as we become older.

Being physically active as we age can also help avoid frailty, a condition in which a person is weak and prone to falling. Maintaining muscular mass, balance, and coordination through regular exercise can lower the risk of falls and injuries.

It's crucial to remember that not all forms of exercise are equivalent. Exercise that targets many aspects of fitness, such as cardiovascular fitness, strength, balance, and flexibility, is crucial as we age. Exercises like brisk walking, cycling, swimming, weight training, and yoga can fall under this category.

Recognizing the restrictions and modifications to Pilates for seniors

Pilates is a type of exercise that emphasizes balance improvement, flexibility improvement, and core strengthening. It can be an excellent type of exercise for seniors because it is low-impact and can enhance physical fitness and mobility. To guarantee that elders can practice Pilates safely, however, there may be a few adjustments that are required.

For elders, a few adaptations that can be required include:

1. Using tools to help with balance and stability, such as a chair or a foam roller
2. Adjusting activities to be more difficult or easier depending on the individual's level of fitness
3. Adjusting the range of motion to minimize the risk of injury
4. Adding additional time for rest and recovery in between workouts

Additionally, it's critical to work with a certified Pilates instructor who has expertise in teaching senior citizens and can make any necessary modifications.

CHAPTER 1

Basic Pilates Principles

Control, attention, fluidity, precision, and breathing are among Pilates' core values.

Control is the capacity to direct one's motions and muscular contractions during an exercise. To carry out the exercises correctly and with good form, concentration is the mental focus necessary.

The term "flow" describes the seamless transition between workouts. Precision is the accurate positioning and performance of each movement. Pilates emphasizes the importance of breathing with deep, controlled inhalations and exhalations woven throughout the movements.

Together, these ideas enhance well-being, balance, and general health.

Breathing Techniques

Pilates places a lot of emphasis on breathing exercises since they improve overall muscle function and oxygenate the body. It's crucial to concentrate on safe and simple procedures when working with seniors.

- **Diaphragmatic breathing**: Using this method, you breathe deeply into your abdomen as opposed to your chest. Sit or lie down in a comfortable position and place one hand on the abdomen and the other on the chest to do diaphragmatic breathing. Focus on extending the abdomen as you inhale and contracting it as you exhale as you inhale through the nose and out the mouth, respectively.

- **Breathing when seated**: You can use this method while seated on a mat or a chair. Start by sitting up straight and letting your shoulders down. Focus on expanding the ribcage as you inhale and compressing it as you exhale as you take in the air via the nose and out the mouth.

- **Abdominal Breathing**: Similar to diaphragmatic breathing, abdominal breathing places more attention on tightening the abdominal muscles during exhalation. The core can be strengthened as a result, and posture can be improved.

- **Breathing with pursed lips**: Seniors who struggle to breathe owing to diseases like COPD or emphysema may find this practice helpful. To breathe with pursed lips, inhale through the nose and exhale through the mouth while maintaining a tight seal on the lips as if you were extinguishing a candle.

Position and Alignment

In particular, for seniors, Pilates emphasizes alignment and posture. While good posture helps to increase general balance, flexibility, and strength, proper alignment helps to protect the joints and lower the risk of injury.

Maintaining a neutral spine is crucial to pay attention when performing Pilates exercises. This means that the head, shoulders, and hips should all be in a straight line while maintaining the natural curvature of the spine. To support the lower back, the pelvis should be level and the abdominal muscles should be contracted.

During Pilates exercises, it's important to pay attention to certain alignment areas, such as:

- Shoulders ought to be down and relaxed, away from the ears.
- Lifting the rib cage and widening the chest is necessary.
- The lower back should be supported by contracting the abdominal muscles.

- The pelvis shouldn't be tipped backward or forward; it should be level.
- The feet should be parallel and the knees should be directly over the ankles.
- In Pilates, posture is also significant since it enhances stability, balance, and general body awareness. Seniors with good posture walk more comfortably and with less pain, which lowers their chance of falling.

Maintaining a tall, stretched spine, with the head held high and the shoulders relaxed is crucial when performing Pilates. To support the lower back, the abdominal muscles should be contracted, and the pelvis should be level.

During Pilates exercises, it's important to pay particular attention to the following postural issues:

- The chin should be parallel to the floor and the head held high.
- The shoulders ought to be down, intense, and away from the ears.
- The rib cage should be elevated and the chest should be open.
- The lower back should be supported by contracting the abdominal muscles.
- Hips should be square, and the pelvis should be level.

Pilates is a low-impact form of exercise, making it a wonderful choice for seniors, persons with injuries, or those who have ongoing medical concerns.

Concentration and Centering

Pilates is a type of exercise that places a strong emphasis on controlled movement, perfect alignment, and core strength. Because Pilates helps enhance balance, flexibility, and general physical fitness, it may be advantageous for elders.

Pilates focuses on engaging and developing the core muscles (the muscles of the belly, lower back, and hips) to build a solid foundation for movement, which is one of its key principles. Seniors can benefit from improved balance, better posture, and a lower chance of injury by doing it.

Another crucial element of pilates is the focus. Instead of letting the mind wander, it means to be completely present and concentrated on the exercise and the muscles being used. Seniors can better engage the right muscles and carry out the exercises correctly and securely thanks to this.

To gain strength and enhance balance, seniors must start with a simplified Pilates program and progressively increase the level of difficulty. To make sure they are completing the exercises correctly and safely, they should also seek the advice of a certified Pilates teacher or physical therapist.

In conclusion, seniors may benefit much from Pilates since it can enhance their physical fitness, flexibility, and balance. Seniors who practice Pilates can benefit from its focus and centering techniques, which can help them use the right muscles and do the movements correctly and securely. As they gain strength and improve their balance, they should begin with a modified Pilates exercise and gradually up the challenge.

CHAPTER 2

Pilates Mat Work

Instead of using specific apparatus like the reformer or the Cadillac, Pilates mat work is a sort of Pilates exercise that is performed on a mat. These exercises are a terrific approach to increasing flexibility, strength, and balance and may be performed at home or in a studio.

Breathing, attention, control, precision, and flow are among the foundational concepts of Pilates mat exercises. The "powerhouse" muscles in the deep abdomen region are the focus of the low-impact exercises. This enhances general body awareness, alignment, and posture.

The warm-up exercises in a typical Pilates mat class, like the "hundred" or the "roll-up," are meant to engage the core muscles and get the body ready for the workout. The class will then move on to a range of exercises that focus on various body parts, including the back, arms, and legs. The plank, the bridge, and the leg circles are some of these exercises.

The fact that Pilates mat activity is appropriate for people of various fitness levels and abilities is one of its advantages. Depending on the demands of the person, the exercises can be changed to be either more difficult or less rigorous. Pilates mat exercises are also a low-impact form of physical activity, making them a fantastic alternative for those who have injuries or medical conditions that could prevent them from engaging in more high-impact activities.

In conclusion, Pilates mat work is a fantastic approach to increasing general health and fitness. It places a heavy emphasis on optimal breathing, core muscle attention, balance, control, and precision in movement, all of which can result in a body that is stronger, more flexible, and more balanced. It is a low-impact, adaptive kind of exercise that is a great choice for anyone trying to enhance their physical health and well-being because it can be performed by people of all fitness levels.

Basic Mat Exercises

For elders, try these simple mat exercises:

The Bridge

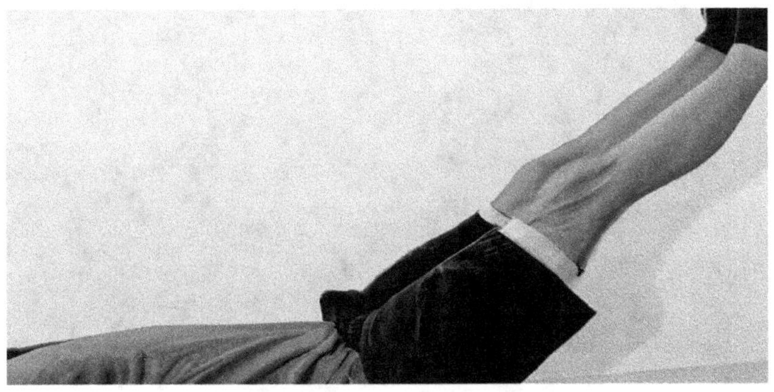

Lie flat on your back with your feet flat on the ground and your knees bent.
Squeeze your glutes at the apex of the movement as you slowly pull your hips upward.
Returning to the initial posture, lower your hips.

- **10-15 times, repeat.**

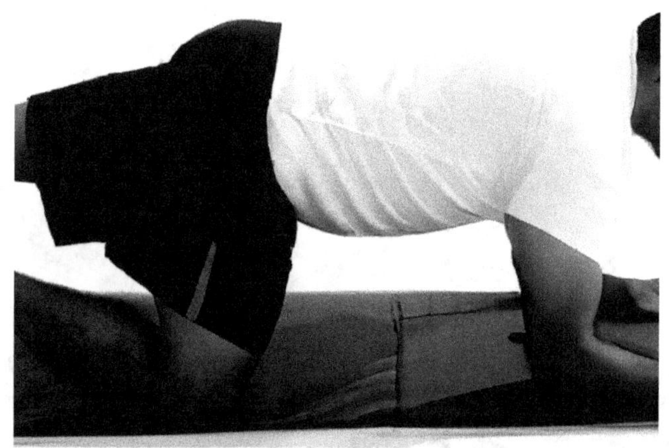

Starting on your hands and knees, place your wrists under your shoulders and your knees under your hips to perform the Cat-Cow position. To do the "cat" part of the workout, arch your back and tuck your chin to your chest. The "cow" element of the exercise is then performed by letting go of your back and lifting your head. 10-15 times, repeat.

The plank

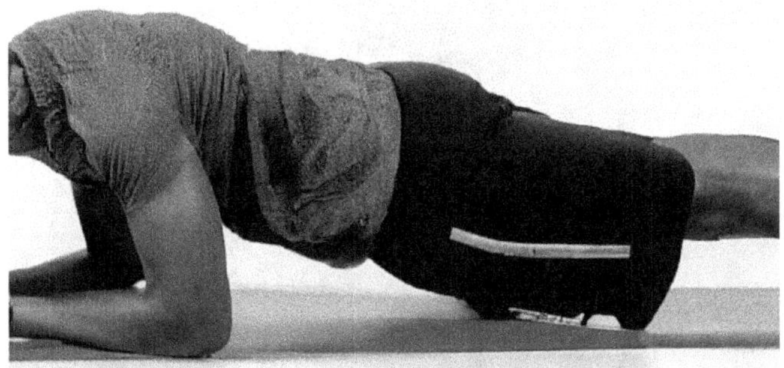

Begin with your feet hip-width apart and your hands and toes under your shoulders. Hold the position for 20 to 30 seconds while maintaining a straight body. Repeat two to three times.

Side plank

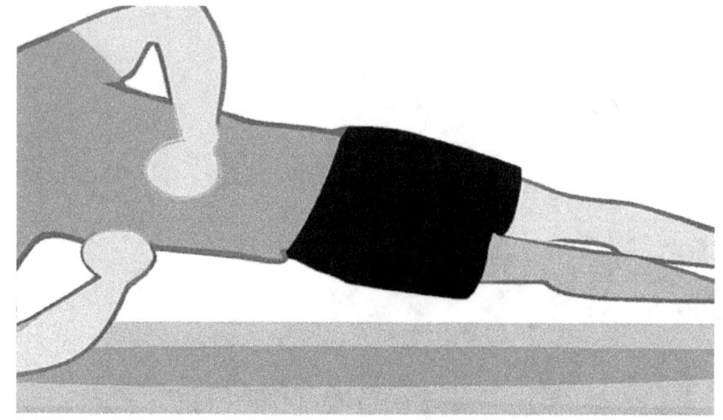

Lay on your side with your feet stacked on top of one another and perform a side plank. By using your elbow as support, elevate your hips off the ground. Hold for 20 to 30 seconds, then alternate sides and do it again.

Leg Raise

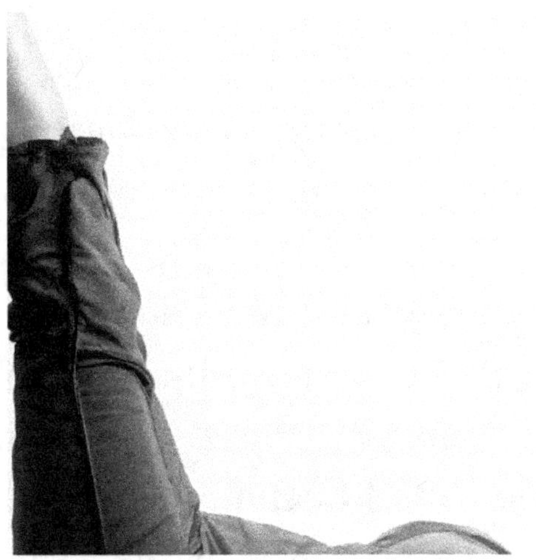

Lay on your back with your legs straight and your arms by your sides to perform the leg raise. One leg should be raised and then slowly brought back down. Before switching legs, repeat for 10 to 15 reps.

Before beginning any workout program, it is imperative to speak with a doctor, especially if you have any medical issues. Additionally, to prevent injury when practicing exercises, always employ proper form and technique.

Modifications for Various Skill Levels

The following modifications for various skill levels are possible during Pilates mat work:

- Beginner adjustments: People who are new to Pilates or have limited mobility often employ these adjustments. Beginner modifications may include completing exercises while seated or lying down, using a thicker mat for increased padding, and leaning against a wall or chair for support.

- Intermediate modifications: People who have strengthened and more flexible and who have a solid understanding of the fundamental Pilates exercises often utilize these modifications. A Pilates ring or ball can be used as a tiny prop, and more challenging exercises like roll-ups and leg circles can be incorporated as intermediate adaptations.

- Advanced adjustments: People who have a high level of strength, flexibility, and endurance and have mastered the fundamental Pilates exercises often employ these modifications. Utilizing more challenging equipment, such as a Pilates reformer or Cadillac, and including exercises like the swan and the teaser are examples of advanced modifications.

To guarantee perfect form and prevent injury, modifications should always be performed under the supervision of a certified Pilates instructor. Additionally, adjustments ought to be changed following each person's unique requirements and capabilities.

Progressions for Increasing Difficulty

- Warm up the muscles and joints by starting with simple movements like knee rolls and leg circles.

- Continue core-strengthening activities like the single-leg stretch and double-leg stretch.

- Include balance and stability-building exercises like the single-leg kick and double-leg kick.

- Continue with leg and hip-strengthening exercises like the bridge and single-leg bridge.

- Introduce exercises that target the arms and shoulders, like the chest rise and roll-up, as the senior gains confidence and comfort with them.

- To increase difficulty and intensity, gradually increase the number of repetitions and sets for each exercise.

- Always be mindful of your posture, your breathing, and your body's signals. If necessary, lessen the exercise's intensity and make the necessary adjustments.

- Before beginning any workout program, it is wise to speak with a healthcare provider, it is crucial to mention.

CHAPTER 3

Introduction to Reformer Pilates

A piece of apparatus used in Pilates workouts is the Pilates Reformer. The Reformer has a sliding carriage, spring-adjustable resistance, and handles and straps for a variety of workouts.

The Reformer is a flexible instrument for strengthening, toning, and stretching the entire body because it provides a wide variety of workouts and resistance levels. It is frequently employed in physical therapy offices and Pilates facilities to strengthen the core, promote posture, and increase flexibility.

Due to the additional resistance and movement of the carriage, some people can find using the Reformer to be more difficult than performing Pilates exercises on a mat. But with the right guidance and adjustments, using the Reformer may be a secure and efficient approach to enhance general health and fitness.

Reformer Pilates Exercises

Standing footwork:

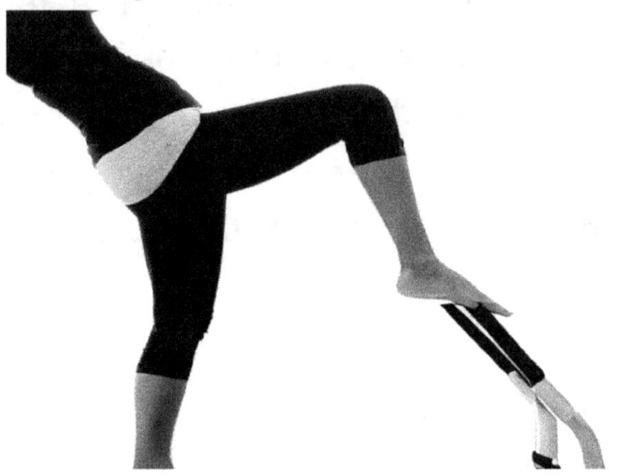

Stand with your feet hip-width apart, engage your core muscles, and keep your spine tall and neutral.

Step one foot back, keeping your weight evenly distributed between both feet.

Bend your front knee to lower your body, keeping your back leg straight.

Push through the heel of your front foot to straighten your leg and return to the starting position.

Repeat the movement on the other leg.

You can add variations by adding arm movement or by making the move more complex by adding a twist or a balance challenge.

Precautions:

As you gain familiarity and confidence, start with simple techniques and progressively raise the challenge.

To prevent putting any muscles or joints under strain, be aware of your posture and form.

Benefits:

1. Balance and coordination are enhanced
2. Increases endurance and leg strength
3. Improves agility and body control
4. Increases concentration and focus.
5. Can aid in keeping elderly folks from falling.
6. Might be a fun and enjoyable approach to getting fitter.

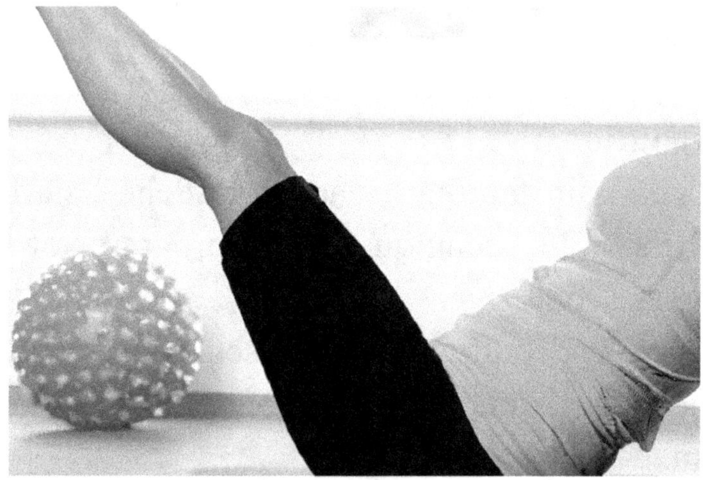

Start in a seated position on the mat with your legs extended in front of you.

Bend your right knee and bring your heel towards your hip.

Use your left hand to hold your right ankle and your right hand to hold your right knee.

Keep your back straight and your core engaged as you gently press your right knee towards the floor.

Hold the stretch for several deep breaths before releasing and repeating on the other leg.

Duration: Typical knee stretches should be held for 5 to 10 seconds at a time.

Precautions:
 A physical therapist should be consulted before performing this exercise if you have knee pain or an injury.

Benefits: Knee stretches can increase joint flexibility and range of motion while also reducing knee pain brought on by tight muscles and tendons.

Leg press:

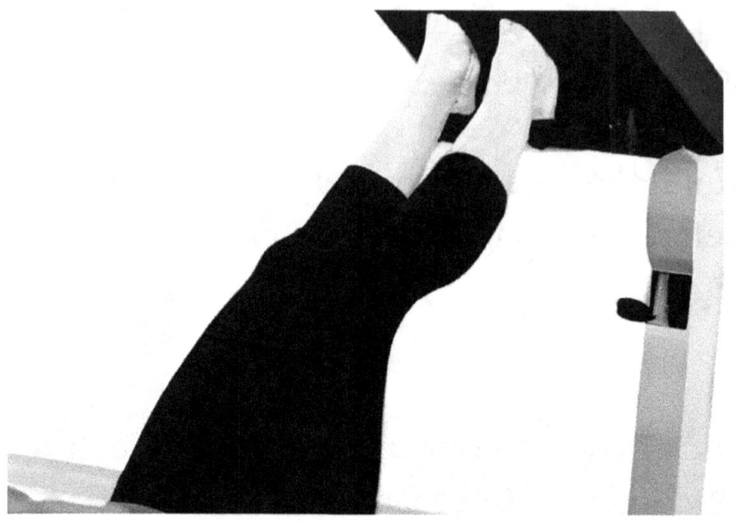

Start in a seated position on the mat with your legs extended in front of you.

Bend your right knee and bring your heel towards your hip.

Use your left hand to hold your right ankle and your right hand to hold your right knee.

Keep your back straight and your core engaged as you gently press your right knee towards the floor.

Hold the stretch for several deep breaths before releasing and repeating on the other leg.

Duration:
An ordinary leg press exercise should be performed for 1-3 sets of 8–12 repetitions.

Precautions: People who have knee or back issues should either stay away from this exercise or only do it with a physical therapist's supervision.

Benefits: Leg presses can increase leg strength and muscle mass while also enhancing general fitness and cardiovascular health.

Arm pull

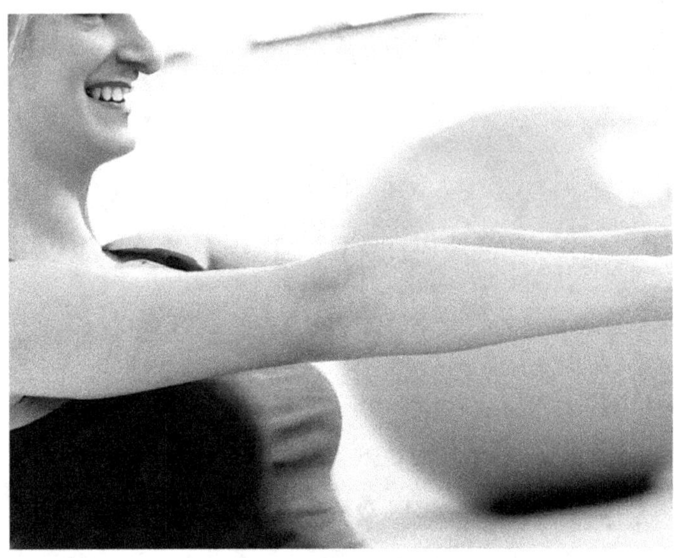

Start in a seated position with your legs in a V shape and your heels together. Your back should be straight and your core engaged.

Reach your arms straight out in front of you, with your palms facing down.

Slowly pull your arms back, keeping them straight and close to your body. Your shoulder blades should come together as you pull your arms back.

Hold the position for a moment, then slowly release your arms back to the starting position.

Duration: An arm pull exercise should be performed for 1-3 sets of 8–12 repetitions.

Precautions:
A physical therapist should be consulted before performing this exercise if you have shoulder pain or an injury.

Benefits: Arm pulls can assist improve posture and general fitness while strengthening the arms, shoulders, and back muscles.

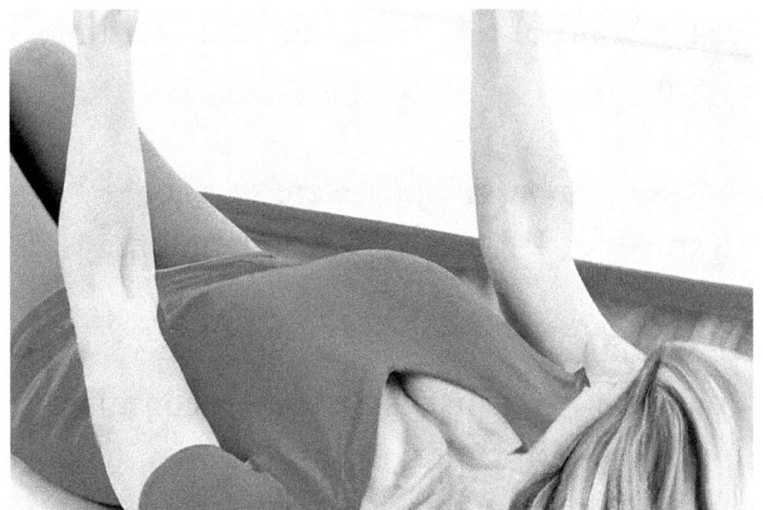

Lay on your back on a mat, with your knees bent and feet flat on the floor. You then raise your head, shoulders, and upper back off the mat, and press your hands together in front of your chest..

Duration:
Typically, 1-3 sets of 8–12 reps should be performed during a chest press exercise.

Precautions:

A physical therapist should be consulted before performing this exercise if you have shoulder pain or an injury.

Benefits:
Chest presses can assist improve posture and general fitness while strengthening the chest, shoulders, and triceps muscles.

Abdominal press

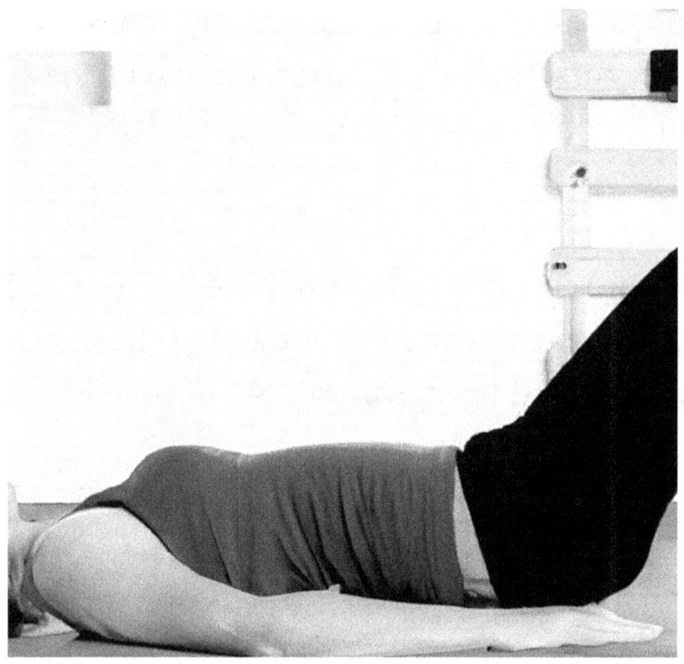

start by lying on your back with your knees bent and your feet flat on the floor. Place your hands behind your head with your elbows out to the sides. Slowly lift your head, shoulders, and upper back off the floor, using your abdominal muscles to press your lower back into the floor. Hold for a count of two, and then slowly lower yourself back down to the starting position. Repeat for several repetitions.

Duration

Regular abdominal press exercises should be performed for 1-3 sets of 8–12 repetitions.

Precautions:

People who have lower back discomfort or injuries should either avoid performing this exercise or do it under the supervision of a physical therapist.

Benefits:

Doing abdominal presses helps enhance posture and general fitness while strengthening and massing the abdominal muscles.

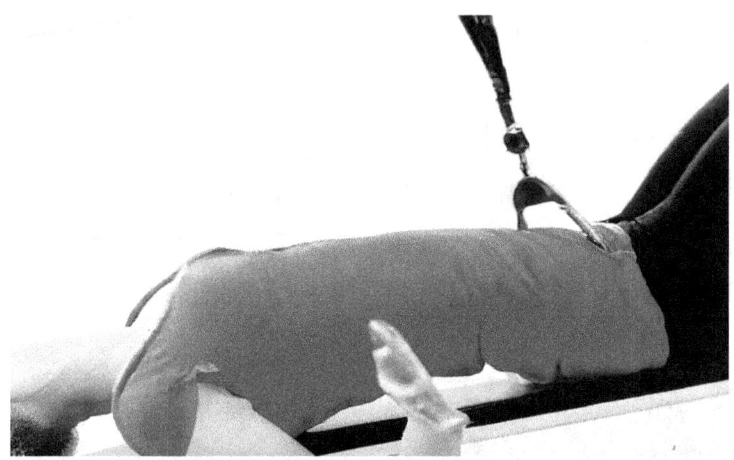

lay on your stomach with the arms stretched out in front of the body. then lifts your head, shoulders, and legs off the mat, using your back muscles to create an arch in the spine

Duration:

 2 to 3 sets of 10 to 15 reps.

Avoid it if you have lower back pain or a recent injury.

Benefits

 include better posture, stronger lower back muscles, and a decreased risk of back problems.

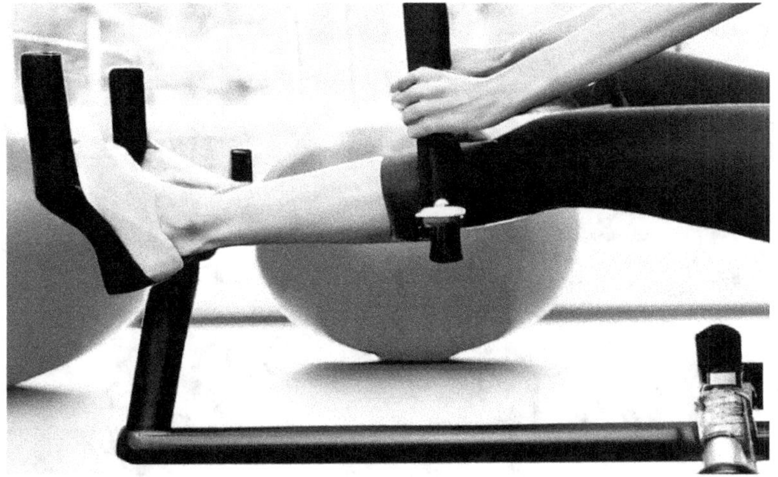

Sit with your legs tucked under the padded lever and then curl your legs up towards your buttocks.

Duration:
2 to 3 sets of 10 to 15 reps.

Precautions
Avoid if you have any knee pain or an injury. Strengthens hamstring muscles, enhances knee stability, and aids in preventing knee problems.

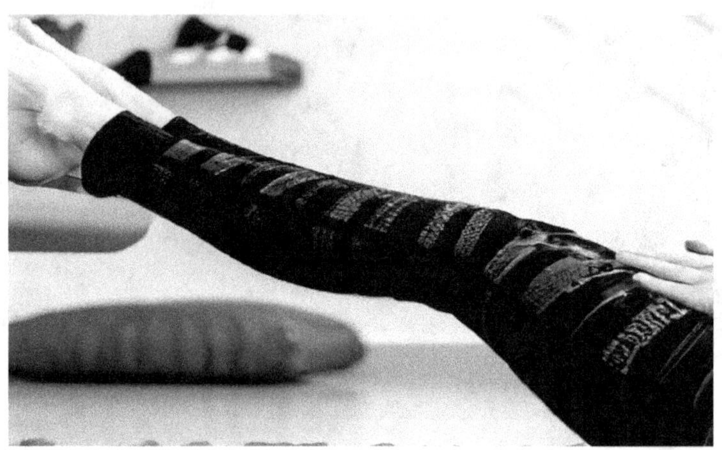

Seated on a Pilates reformer or chair, with your legs extended straight out in front of the body. Bends the knees and extends them back out again, using your thigh muscles to control the movement.

Duration:

2 to 3 sets of 10 to 15 reps.

Avoid if you have any knee pain or an injury.

Benefits include strengthening the quadriceps muscles, increasing knee stability, and reducing the risk of a knee injury.

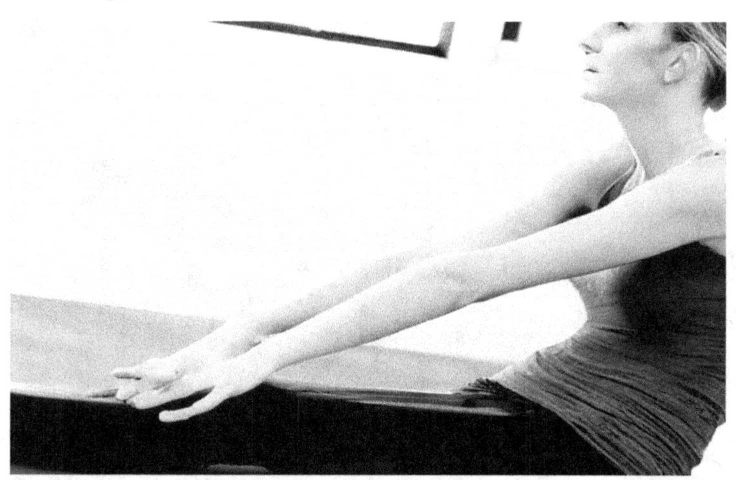

Seat on a mat with your legs extended straight out in front of the body, and the arms reaching out in front with a resistance band or towel.

Duration: 2 to 3 sets of 10 to 15 reps.
Avoid it if you have lower back pain or a recent injury.

Benefits:
Strengthens the upper back muscles and enhances posture.

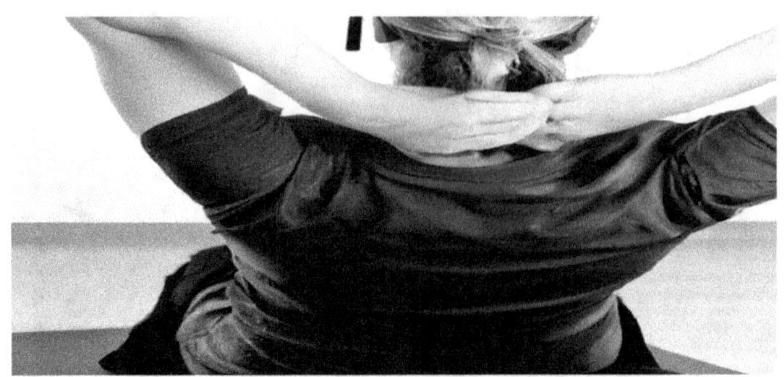

Sit on the edge of a mat or bench with your feet flat on the floor. Hold a weight in each hand, with your elbows bent and hands at shoulder level. Slowly press the weights overhead, straightening your arms, and then lower them back to the starting position. Keep your core engaged and avoid arching your back during the exercise.

Duration: 2 to 3 sets of 10 to 15 reps.

Avoid if you have shoulder discomfort or an injury.

Benefits include improved posture and shoulder muscle strength.

Progression and Modifications

Pilates is a type of exercise that emphasizes developing balance, flexibility, and strength in the midsection. It was created by Joseph Pilates at the beginning of the 20th century, and today individuals of all ages, including seniors, utilize it frequently.

The range of motion in Pilates exercises can be changed to account for any physical restrictions, or they can be modified to use props like a chair or a wall for support. Progressions may entail escalating the level of difficulty or complexity of the workout as the person's flexibility and strength develop over time.

Senior-friendly alteration examples include:
Using a chair or a wall as support when performing exercises like the "hundred" or "roll-ups"
Leg circles and arm work exercises with a lighter resistance band or tiny ball
adjusting exercises like "the plank" so that they are performed on the knees rather than in the full plank position
Senior-specific advancement examples include:

- Gradually upping the number of reps or sets in a workout
- Exercises like "leg lifts" or "arm circles" can be improved by adding tiny weights or resistance bands.
- As the person's strength and flexibility increase, adding more challenging exercises like "the swan" or "the teaser"

CHAPTER 4

Pilates chair work

Pilates Chair Work is a method of workout that makes use of a little, portable chair with a variety of resistance springs, commonly referred to as Wunda Chair exercises. The chair is made to boost general body awareness, flexibility, and core strength.

The exercises done on the chair emphasize modest, controlled motions that work the body's deep muscles, especially the glutes and core. Additionally, the chair permits a broader variety of workouts and variations, making it appropriate for users of all fitness levels.

Exercises like Pilates Chair Work, which are difficult but low-impact, can aid with balance, posture, and general fitness.

Chair workouts

Twist while seated

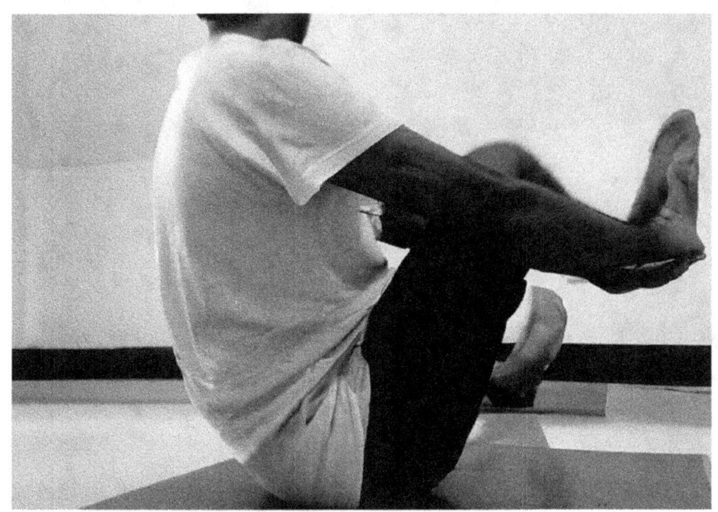

Place your feet flat on the ground and sit tall on the chair. Turn your torso to the right while placing your left hand on your right knee.

Hold for two to three seconds before performing 10-15 repetitions of each side. Benefits: This workout increases torso flexibility.

Sitting Leg Extension:

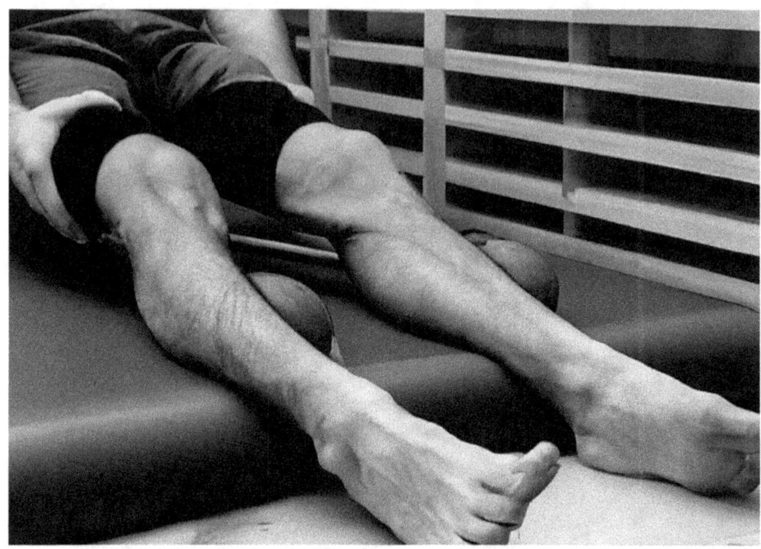

Place your feet flat on the floor while sitting tall in the chair. One leg out in front of you should be slowly straightened before being brought back to the starting position.

Repeat on each leg 10 to 15 times total.
The quadriceps are strengthened by this exercise.

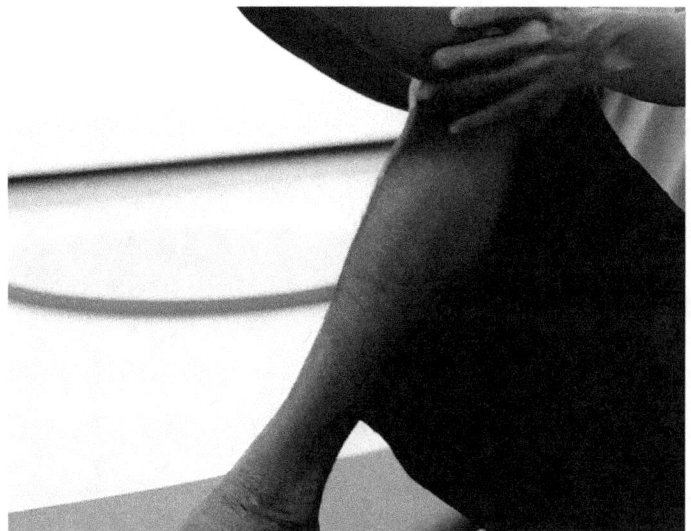

Place your feet firmly on the ground while sitting tall in the chair. One leg should be slowly rotating in a clockwise direction.

15 to 20 repetitions total, then repeat in a clockwise motion.

Benefit: This exercise increases hip and leg flexibility.

Seated Cat-Cow

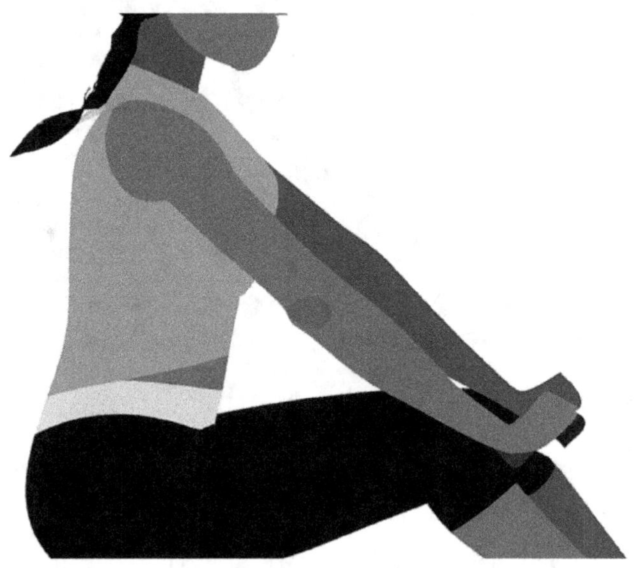

Place your feet flat on the ground while sitting tall in the chair. Lift your head, arch your back, let go, and tuck your chin into your chest.

Repeat for 10 to 15 times total.

Benefit: The spine's flexibility is improved by this workout.

Seated Spinal Extension

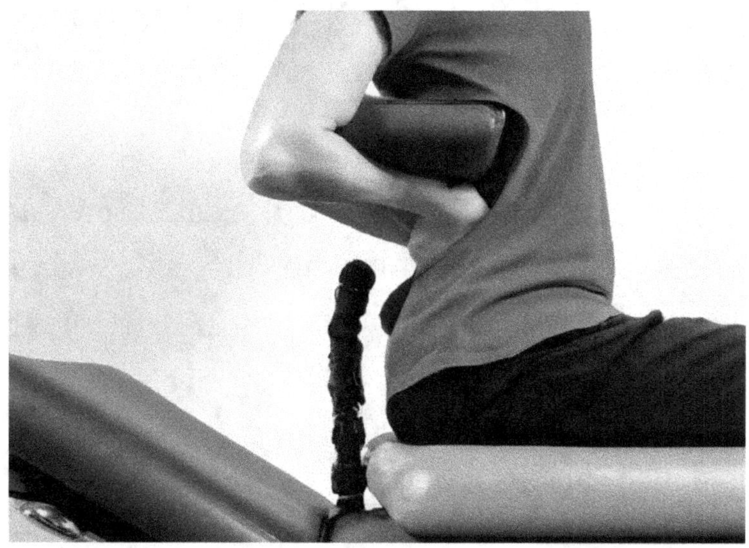

Sit tall on the chair with your feet flat on the floor. Lean back, put your hands on the back of your head, then let go and sit up straight. Repeat ten to fifteen times. The upper back muscles are strengthened by this workout.

Progression and Modifications

Single Leg Extension: When performing the exercise, elevate one leg off the chair and stretch it straight out in front of you.

Oblique Rotate: While still seated on the chair, twist your torso to the side while working your oblique muscles.

Pilates Chair for Standing: Use the chair for balance and support while performing the workout while standing as opposed to sitting.

Pilates Chair in Reverse: While executing the exercise in the reverse posture, face the back of the chair and lean on it for support.

Resistance bands can be used in the Pilates chair exercise to increase the intensity and challenge the muscles.

Holding tiny weights in your hands as you perform the Pilates chair exercise will add resistance and improve muscle tone.

Pilates Chair with a Ball: To strengthen your core and enhance balance while executing the exercise, sit on a stability ball rather than a chair.

Pilates Chair with a Step: To enhance your range of motion and challenge your legs, use a step or bench to elevate your feet while executing the exercise.

Special Considerations for Seniors

Painful joints and arthriti

Seniors with arthritis and joint pain may benefit from the Pilates exercise method. However, it's crucial to bear the following in mind when creating a Pilates program for this group:

Exercises in Pilates can be changed to account for arthritis and joint pain. Exercises can be performed, for instance, while seated or with the use of accessories like resistance bands or chairs.

Low-impact: Because Pilates has a low impact on the joints, it is a good workout for seniors with arthritis and joint pain.

Strengthening: Pilates places a strong emphasis on stabilizing muscles and the core, which can support and safeguard the joints.

Flexibility: Pilates also increases your range of motion and flexibility, which can assist to lessen joint discomfort and stiffness.

Consultation: Before beginning a Pilates program, speak with a physiotherapist or a doctor, especially if you have any medical conditions or are taking any drugs that can limit your ability to exercise.

Movements in Pilates are slow and controlled, which can assist seniors in becoming aware of their bodies, moving correctly, and preventing injuries.

Pay attention to pain: If an elderly person feels pain while performing a Pilates exercise, they should stop and seek medical advice.

To make the session safe and enjoyable, Pilates can be modified to the student's requirements and skills.

In conclusion, seniors with arthritis and joint discomfort may find Pilates to be a helpful type of exercise, but adaptations and safety measures must be implemented. It is advised to consult a healthcare expert.

Bone health and Osteoporosis

Osteoporosis is a disease that weakens and brutalizes the bones. It is a frequent problem in older people and it can make fractures and other types of injuries more likely. Pilates is a type of exercise that can benefit elderly people with osteoporosis bone health.

Pilates has a strong emphasis on the core muscles, which enhances stability and balance. Seniors with osteoporosis may experience fewer fractures and fall as a result of this. Push-ups and arm circles are two upper body movements included in pilates that can help to build bone density in the arms and shoulders.

Pilates can also help seniors with osteoporosis lower their risk of falls and fractures by enhancing their flexibility, coordination, and posture.

To ensure safety, a healthcare professional can assist in choosing the right workouts and making any required modifications.

A good diet and various forms of exercise, along with Pilates, can assist to improve general bone health, but Pilates by itself is insufficient to prevent and treat osteoporosis.

Balance and prevention from falling

It targets the muscles that support the spine, hips, and shoulders, which helps to improve balance and prevent falls. Pilates movements are done with control and precision, which enhances proprioception (the capacity to perceive one's body's position in space) and neuromuscular control.

Here are several Pilates moves that can improve balance and decrease fall risk:

Standing on one leg while lifting the other one off the ground is known as single-leg balancing. This helps to strengthen the muscles in the legs and hips and enhance balance.

Lying on your back while doing this exercise requires you to elevate your hips toward the ceiling. Balance is improved and the core muscles are strengthened during this activity.

With your arms straight and your body in a straight line, you must hold your body in a push-up position as you perform the plank exercise. Balance is improved and the core muscles are strengthened during this activity.

The Saw: For this exercise, sit with your legs wide apart and touch your toes with your forward reach. This practice helps to increase balance and flexibility.

The roll-up is a workout that entails lying on your back, raising your head, shoulders, and legs off the ground, and then rolling up to a seated position. This practice enhances balance while strengthening the core muscles.

It is significant to remember that maintaining balance and preventing falls should be a priority for seniors and anybody else who may be at risk for falling.

Advice on how to design your Pilates routine

To ascertain your level of fitness and any unique requirements or limits, speak with a Pilates instructor or physical therapist.
Set attainable objectives for yourself, such as gaining core strength or more flexibility.
Start with simple exercises and build up your comfort and confidence before moving on to more complex workouts.
Mix in some mat exercises like the Hundred and the Roll-Up as well as workouts using machines like the Reformer and the Cadillac.
To optimize the advantages of each exercise and avoid injury, pay close attention to good form and alignment.
Throughout each exercise, be careful to breathe evenly and deeply.
To get a well-rounded workout, mix up your regimen with both aerobic and strength-training routines.

Include stretches and relaxation techniques, like Savasana, to reduce stress and increase flexibility.

Avoid boredom by mixing up your routine and keeping your body engaged.

Pay attention to your body and modify the time and intensity of your workout as necessary.

Aim for at least three times a week of regular practice.

Do not forget to enjoy yourself and the process!

Monitoring progress and taking safety precautions

Strength, flexibility, balance, and general physical function can all be measured as progress is made throughout a senior Pilates session. This can be accomplished by routine evaluations that include gauging range of motion, muscular strength, and overall mobility.

Seniors who practice Pilates should take extra care to follow safety precautions, which may include altering the exercises to lower the risk of injury, using props like mats, blocks, and straps to provide support and stability, and working with a qualified instructor who is experienced working with seniors and their unique needs. Additionally, it's crucial to ensure that seniors are not in pain or discomfort while performing the exercises and to make any necessary adjustments to account for any physical restrictions.

The benefits of regular Pilates practice for seniors

Pilates is a type of exercise that has numerous advantages for seniors. The following are a few advantages:

Improved flexibility and balance are possible thanks to Pilates, which emphasizes controlled movements and breathing.

Muscles in the core are strengthened, which can help seniors maintain excellent posture and lower their risk of falling. Pilates places a strong emphasis on this.

Low impact: Pilates is a low-impact form of physical activity, making it a wonderful choice for seniors who might experience joint pain or other restrictions.

Pilates places a strong emphasis on relaxation and mindfulness, which can help lower stress and enhance mental health.

Improved Bone Density: As people age, it's crucial to maintain bone density, which Pilates has been shown to do.

Conclusion

Seniors who do Pilates may find it helpful. Flexibility, balance, and core strength can all be enhanced by it. Additionally, because it has a mild impact, it is a suitable choice for people who have joint problems or other physical restrictions. Before beginning any new workout program, you should always speak with your doctor, especially if you have any health issues or concerns.

Encouragement to maintain an active, healthy lifestyle

The key to general well-being is to stay active and lead a healthy lifestyle. Regular exercise can lower the chance of developing chronic diseases including obesity, type 2 diabetes, and heart disease, build bones and muscles, and enhance cardiovascular health. You may also provide your body with the nutrients it needs by eating a balanced diet that is high in fruits, vegetables, whole grains, and lean protein. It's crucial to strike a balance between physical activity and enough relaxation. Set reasonable objectives and recognize tiny accomplishments along the way. You might also try to include enjoyable things in your daily schedule. Consistency is crucial; develop the habit of making good decisions.

Glossary

A lexicon of some Pilates words is provided below:

The term "core" describes the muscles in the lower back, hips, trunk, and torso.

Joseph Pilates' original term for the Pilates method was Contrology.

Exercises performed on a mat without the use of equipment are called mat work.

A piece of workout equipment called a reformer employs straps and springs to produce resistance for exercises.

The process of centering involves contracting the abdominal muscles and focusing attention on the body's center.

The smooth, fluid movement used in Pilates movements is referred to as "flow."

Precision in Pilates movements refers to the emphasis on precise alignment and form.

Senior Pilates Exercise Plan

- **Warm-Up (5 minutes):**

1. Gentle Neck Tilts:

   - Sit or stand comfortably, slowly tilt your head side to side for 1 minute.

2. Shoulder Rolls:

   - Roll your shoulders forward and backward in a smooth motion for 2 minutes.

3. Deep Breathing:

   - Inhale deeply through your nose, exhale through your mouth. Focus on filling and emptying your lungs completely for 2 minutes.

- **Pilates Routine (20 minutes):**

4. Pelvic Tilts:
   - Lie on your back, bend knees, and engage your core. Lift your pelvis slightly, hold, and lower. Repeat for 2 sets of 10.

5. Leg Circles:
   - Lie on your back, extend one leg, and draw small circles in the air. Switch legs after 10 circles. Repeat for 2 sets.

6. Seated Spine Twist:
   - Sit tall in a chair, twist your torso gently to one side, hold, and return to center. Repeat on the other side. Perform 2 sets of 12 twists.

7. Modified Side Plank:
   - From a side-lying position, prop yourself up on your elbow, keeping your knees bent. Hold for 20 seconds each side, repeat twice.

8. Bridge Exercise:

- Lie on your back, lift your hips toward the ceiling, engaging your glutes and core. Hold for 15 seconds, lower, and repeat for 2 sets of 10.

9. Seated Leg Lifts:

- Sit on the edge of a chair, lift one leg straight in front of you, hold, and lower. Switch legs after 10 lifts. Perform 2 sets.

10. Pilates Swimming:

- Lie on your stomach, lift your opposite arm and leg simultaneously, then switch. Repeat for 2 sets of 12.

- **Cool Down (5 minutes):**

11. Child's Pose:

- Kneel on the floor, sit back on your heels, and stretch your arms forward. Hold for 2 minutes, focusing on deep breaths.

12. Seated Forward Bend:

- Sit with legs extended, hinge at your hips, and reach toward your toes. Hold for 2 minutes, breathing deeply.

13. Neck and Shoulder Stretch:

- Gently tilt your head to one side, bringing your ear toward your shoulder. Hold for 30 seconds each side.

- **Tips:**
- Perform these exercises on a comfortable mat or carpet.
- Start with 10 minutes and gradually increase the duration as you become more comfortable.
- Listen to your body, and if any exercise causes discomfort, skip or modify it.
- Consult with a healthcare professional before starting any new exercise routine.

Always prioritize safety and enjoy the benefits of Pilates for improved strength, flexibility, and overall well-being.

Scan this Area to access bonus